Table of Contents

Detoxifying the body has become an clear key preventative measure to numerous types of health problems. Since most of us are busy, and unable or unwilling to keep a strict diet in request to completely eliminate all the toxins from our body. We have chemicals building up in our bodies day after day. Since these synthetics are not unsafe in little amounts, only in larger accumulated amounts, we don't notice side effects until we are much older. A proper, even if occasional, detox diet is necessary to relieve our bodies of harmful toxins and chemicals, and keep a healthy, normal, and seemingly perpetual life. The primary idea of a detox diet is to wipe out almost all foods and restrict the body to only water and vegetables for a couple days; usually around 5 or 6 days is adequate. Most detox consumes less calories at that point permit for a sluggish re-presentation of other foods, gradually. The eats less for the most part confine foods from your diet that are said to have unsafe toxins. Along with this a detox diet should then flush the current poisons out of the body. A detox diet basically gives the liver and other organs a chance to get up and remove all the toxins. This is done through our sweat, feces, and urine. Our bodies just cannot adapt to the normal day to day ingestion of synthetic compounds. Most these chemicals come from food sources, as mentioned previously, yet also have a wide variety of other sources. Despite the fact that we do not know what foods are the cause of it all, we do know that pesticides, heavy metals, such as mercury and lead, and the chemicals in cigarettes and the air we breath, all enter our bodys via our lungs or stomach and can cause an excessive build up. These synthetic compounds in small amounts are harmless; its the day after day ingestion and develop of them which can lead to degenerative sicknesses. One common detox diet is the combination of nothing however fruits and water for a given period. The advancement of chemicals being metabolized by our bodies can be helped with certain vitamins, herbs and supplements. A few enhancements will help the assembly of toxins in our fat and other toxin deposits found throughout the body. Since our bodies free themselves of chemicals through sweat, sauna treatments can likewise provide a great benefit. There are numerous other diets and detox treatments, these are just a couple common strategies. Normal body detoxification is a good preventative action and advances a better present and future!You know there are certain people who go into detox in order to rid themselves of certain addictions. When in reference to a diet, it can mean the same thing. Detox is a shortened adaptation of the word "detoxification," which is a term that means the elimination of toxins from the body. The detox diet basically means that you're eliminating poisons from your bloodstream, liver, kidneys and intestines by methods for an exacting eating regimen. The detox diet has a purpose beyond basically ridding your body of poisons. True, "toxin," as a word with all its connotations, sounds horrible. Yet, the belief that fuels the detox diet is that all these toxins we take in and ingest everyday cause skin problems, headaches, fatigue and sickness. The goal of the detox diet is to help get the body back to a healthful, new state. The elimination of the toxins is believed to purify the body and help it work better.The notion of a detox diet wasn't invented in this decade. It's been around for quite a long time, and several cultures throughout history have lauded the effects of detoxification. Generally, a detox diet can be summed up as a low-calorie, primarily liquid diet that has the goal of cleansing the body. Though there are several detox diets with diverse explicit plans, such as the Fruit Flush and Martha's Vineyard Detox Diet, the general idea behind them all is the same.

Let's face it. Western medicine has (and is) failing us. A more recent analysis estimates 128,000 Americans die each year as a result of taking medications as prescribed – or nearly five times the number of people killed by overdosing on prescription painkillers and heroin, according to US News. Detoxification was (and is) a key component of its methods, reminding us again that toxins have been a known problem from the very beginning of medicine and healing. Ancient Biblical regulations for life and for temple activity include dietary restrictions, physical cleansing and aromatic cleansing. Detoxification is an ancient process that dates back as far as the Roman, Greek, Native American and Indian Cultures. The premise surrounds around the process of purification and cleansing. Many effective techniques are still sound ways to rid the body of toxins.

Detoxification, or detox, generally refers to the process of removing toxins from the body. In the case of substance use, detox specifically refers to the period of time that the body is allowed to process or metabolize any unnaturally foreign substance in the system and, in doing so, clears their toxic influence. Basically, detoxification means cleansing the blood. This is done by removing impurities from the blood in the liver, where toxins are processed for elimination. The body also eliminates toxins through the kidneys, intestines, lungs, lymphatic system, and skin

What Is a Detox?

Depending on who you ask, the detox diet meaning can vary pretty widely. For some, it may be considered an intense cleansing diet that consists of drinking strange concoctions for weeks on end to clear out toxins and achieve weight loss. For others, the term "detox cleanse" is little more than a marketing ploy used to shill expensive and overpriced products to health-conscious consumers. In reality, a detox diet can be a healthy way to get back on track and help your body do exactly what it's designed to do: clear out toxins and keep you in tip-top shape. See, your body has a complex detox system built right in, and all of your organs work together to keep you feeling healthy. Your skin pushes out bacteria through the sweat, your kidneys filter through liters of blood and produce urine, your lungs expel carbon dioxide, your intestines extract nutrients from food to excrete waste products, and your liver clears out toxins from the body. Factors like chronic stress, unhealthy habits, physical inactivity and a diet high in ultra-processed foods can totally tank your body's natural detox system, making it even harder to remove toxins from the bloodstream efficiently. A body cleanse or detox diet that involves cutting out junk foods and increasing your intake of nutritious whole foods along with a few powerful detox foods can be an easy way to help your body detox and hit the reset button. Best of all, unlike on other detox diets, this kind of natural cleanse won't drain your energy levels or leave you feeling worn down. Instead, it can boost energy, restore motivation and help you feel your best.Detox diets are generally short-term dietary interventions designed to eliminate toxins from your body. A typical detox diet involves a period of fasting, followed by a strict diet of fruit, vegetables, fruit juices, and water. Sometimes a detox also includes herbs, teas, supplements, and colon cleanses or enemas.

This is claimed to:

Rest your organs by fasting

Stimulate your liver to get rid of toxins

Promote toxin elimination through feces, urine, and sweat

Provide your body with healthy nutrients

Detox therapies are most commonly recommended because of potential exposure to toxic chemicals in the environment or your diet. These include pollutants, synthetic chemicals, heavy metals, and other harmful compounds. These diets are also claimed to help with various health problems, including obesity, digestive issues, autoimmune diseases, inflammation, allergies, bloating, and chronic fatigue. However, human research on detox diets is lacking, and the handful of studies that exist are significantly flawed.

There are many ways to do a detox diet — ranging from total starvation fasts to simpler food modifications.

Most detox diets involve at least one of the following:

Fasting for 1–3 days.

Drinking fresh fruit and vegetable juices, smoothies, water, and tea.

Drinking only specific liquids, such as salted water or lemon juice.

Eliminating foods high in heavy metals, contaminants, and allergens.

Taking supplements or herbs.

Avoiding all allergenic foods, then slowly reintroducing them.

Using laxatives, colon cleanses, or enemas.

Exercising regularly.

Completely eliminating alcohol, coffee, cigarettes, and refined sugar.

What is a detox diet?

This hustle culture of today may bring in a lot of excitement and rush into a person's life. However; one cannot neglect the poor lifestyle choices that one might make due to this, such as drinking a lot of coffee or eating outside. This fast-paced life can sometimes lead to the negligence of one's health and well-being. It is said that over time, due to poor food choices, exposure to harmful chemicals, and various forms of pollution, several toxins accumulate within the body. A

detox diet aims to remove
unwanted substances present in
the body and also the increase
absorption of vitamins and
minerals. Such a diet generally
consists of drinking a lot of fluids,
eating whole foods, or even fasting
for a few days or sometimes even
a week.

Detox diets vary significantly from each other in terms of practice as well as intensity.

Master Cleanse Diet

In this diet you are supposed to consume a combination of cayenne pepper, lemon juice and maple syrup mixed in water. It is a gentle diet as the maple syrup which is easily absorbed regulates the release of toxins as stored fats, thus converting it to energy gradually.

Juiec Fast

It is another type of liquid detox diet. You are supposed to consume fruit or vegetable juices, or a combination of both. Apart from detoxification, you have the added benefits of enzymes, minerals and vitamins which help to rejuvenate the body. The best part of the diet is that it is easy on your digestive system, as the body can assimilate them directly without the need of any digestive enzymes.

Mono Fruit Detox Diet

The word mono would give you a clue that the diet will consist of only a single type of fruit. The diet can be done for a prolonged period, as the organic water of the fruit allows the body cells to clean themselves. When the water comes out, it takes out along with it harmful toxins. The use of only one fruit also makes your body?s pH more stable, and regulates your sugar level.

Raw Food Detox Diet

Raw foods are eaten to maintain the levels of vitamins, minerals and other essentials. These things are lost when food is cooked or washed. The digestive enzymes present in the raw food also aids metabolism process, and fortifies immunity. The optimum potassium-to-sodium ratio is also maintained, which improves cell functioning and the pH balance thus realizing the objective of a detox diet.

Hallelujah Diet

Many people are not comfortable with the idea of having all meals consisting of only raw food. As an alternative, this diet allows you to eat 85% raw food and 15% cooked food. The only restriction is that the cooked meal can be eaten only at the end of the evening meal. Also, breakfast has to be skipped and only barley grass drinks and fresh vegetable juices can be had instead then. It?ll take some time to get habituated to the regimen of skipping breakfast though if you are used to it. This switch is easier if you replace bacon and eggs with almond milk, fresh fruit salad, and sprouted grain toast with almond butter and whole grain raw granola.

Diuretic Diet

This not only reduces body fat, but also helps the body to release fluids. Certain herbs like asparagus, artichoke, celery seed, dandelion, juniper berries, melon, parsley and watercress assist in this. Some food supplements and beverages like coffee, coke and tea are also diuretics. Only some of the many types of detox diets have been mentioned above. There are many more. If you are not happy with the programs above, then you can search for some other alternatives. But remember to consult your doctor before you start any diet to know whether or not the diet is safe for your health.

Juice or smoothie cleanse

These liquid-only cleanses, which are arguably the most popular, replace solid foods with a selection of fruit- and vegetable-based juices or smoothies. Typically, juice and smoothie cleanses last anywhere between 3 and 21 days — although some people go much longer. There are tons of companies out there that sell these kinds of cleanses. You can also buy juices and smoothies from a specialized shop or make them at home.

Drinking fruit- and vegetable-based juices — as long as they're fresh-pressed — and smoothies can definitely be healthy. These drinks are often packed with nutrients, especially if they go heavy on the veggies, and can be a great addition to your diet. But drinking only juices and smoothies and depriving your body of actual food is where this detox veers into unhealthy territory.

"Typically, [liquid] detoxes remove the majority of protein and fat from the diet," says Reaver.

Not only does the lack of protein and fat mean you'll spend your entire detox feeling hungry, but it can also lead to a host of other negative side effects.

"These detoxes can lead to low blood sugar, brain fog, decreased productivity, and fatigue," Reaver adds.

Liver detox

Another hot trend in the cleanse world is what's called "liver detoxes." The aim of a liver detox is to deliver a boost to the body's detoxifying system by improving liver function. While this sounds like a great idea — it's never a bad idea to eat a diet that supports healthy liver function — you don't need a formal "detox" in order to do so.

"Fortunately, the liver is well-equipped to handle the toxins that we're most commonly exposed to," says Reaver.

"Instead of a 'detox' [...] people should [focus on] eating a diet that's rich in both raw and cooked fruits and vegetables; includes soluble fiber like beans, nuts, and grains; and limits alcohol intake. These are the essential building blocks that'll allow your liver to operate at peak function."

Food restriction

Another form of detox are ones that restrict certain foods or food groups as a way to flush the body of toxins and improve overall health. Restricting or eliminating certain foods in your diet can be helpful under certain circumstances and if you do it the right way.

"Some people benefit from a cleanse because it removes food groups that may cause them discomfort, like gluten or dairy," says Reaver.

The key, however, is to be strategic in your restriction.

"Instead of eliminating most foods, try to remove a type of food for a week and see if you feel better," explains Reaver.

"Then, add the food back in and monitor your symptoms. If bloating, gas, intestinal discomfort, constipation, or diarrhea return, then it may be a good idea to remove that food group from your diet."

However, eliminating too many foods or whole food groups at once, like some food cleanses require you to do, will not only feel overly restrictive, it also won't give you any insight into what foods are negatively impacting your health.

Colon cleanse

Most cleanses attempt to get rid of toxins through dietary changes. But there are also cleanses that attempt to flush the body from the other end. Colon cleanses attempt to cleanse the digestive tract and rid the body of toxins by promoting bowel movements via supplements or laxatives. Colon hydrotherapy, also known as a colonic, removes waste manually by flushing the colon with water. Either way, these cleanses work to remove built-up waste — which they claim will also remove toxins and improve overall health. But not only are colon cleanses extremely unpleasant, but they may also be dangerous.

"Colon cleanses and colon hydrotherapy should be avoided unless done at the direction of a physician," explains Reaver.

"They may cause stomach cramping, diarrhea, and vomiting. More serious outcomes can include bacterial infection, perforated bowels, and electrolyte imbalance that can cause kidney and heart problems."

Instead, Reaver suggests consuming a diet high in soluble and insoluble fiber to help clear out waste.

"These two types of fiber will effectively remove debris and undigested food particles from the colon that can cause bloating, painful excretion, and constipation."

Why should I do a detox diet?

A detox diet has several advantages, physically and mentally. In addition to cleansing the body of toxins, a detox diet also has positive effects on mental health. According to the experiences shared by a number of people who followed this diet, a detox brings about a sense of calm, freshness, and peace within the body. Others have also reported feeling rejuvenated and energized. On a closer look, one can also find instances of fasting in many cultures which are said to bring about this feeling of serenity but also build discipline. Hence, the idea of fasting or limiting diet for specific kinds of food at specific times of the day is not completely alien. These detox diets are mainly used for weight-loss, to decrease consumption of substances like alcohol, tobacco or coffee, to overcome ailments such as headaches or joint pain and even to just improve one's eating habits.

With our fast paced lifestyles, we tend to eat more fast food and less healthy home cooked meals. Fast foods contain a very high fat percentage and very few nutrients. They are often high in fat soluble chemicals that are foreign to your body and gets stored as fat tissue when your liver cannot break it down due to all the toxins it?s already fighting. This results in your body going into slow mode causing you to feel tired, irritated, hormonal and ill. Your skin suffers, your metabolism slows down and you start to look and feel unhealthy. Changing your lifestyle and doing a regular detox, your energy will improve, your skin?s natural glow will return, your concentration will improve and so also your metabolism, increasing your energy and burning fat. Depending on your situation and the state of your health, care should be taken when pregnant or breastfeeding, as a strict detox can be detrimental to the health of the mother and the baby. It?s always a good idea to consult your doctor if you suffer from heart disease, anaemia or any blood related disease, cancer, high/low blood pressure, alcohol dependency syndrome, drug related problems etc.

Important things to know about detoxifying

Side effects commonly occur with the detox process as your body starts to clear itself. This is normal. Drink plenty of water to assist your body in the detoxification process almost like rinsing it clean. Not everyone will experience the same effects while on a detox as our bodies respond in different ways. The first symptom to appear is usually a mild throbbing headache, followed by tiredness as jour body is adjusting to the new routine. A good idea is to start your detox on a Friday to give your body time over the weekend to rest and adjust. Other symptoms include diarrhoea, restlessness and sleeplessness. Unless your detox is a lifestyle change like cutting down on alcohol and cigarette, do not continue for longer than 3 days. Try to cleanse your body three to four times a year with the changes of the season. Before jumping into a really hectic detox, make sure to consult your doctor or health specialist. Read as much as you can about a specific detox diet and avoid not eating at all. Some detox diets can be a really bad experience and do much worse for your health than good. Read reviews about it and make sure you choose the one that?s right for you.

As far as diets go, the detox diet is quite a restrictive one. The diet requires you to give up many foods that have ingredients believed to be toxins. Because it's so restrictive, experts recommend that dieters only rely on the detox plan for a small amount of time. And it's best to make sure you have no pressing health issues that could be complicated by such a rigorous diet. Though there are several detox diets out there, the most basic one involves three days of fasting on water and then 10 days of a monotrophic diet. A monotrophic diet is just a fancy term for limiting yourself to one type of fruit per meal [source: The Diet Channel]. In between lunch and dinner, though, some detox diets do allow a large glass of fresh carrot juice. After following the plan for 13 days, according to this basic type of detox diet, you would then ease into a more normal diet by eating strictly raw food. In addition to the food regimen, some detox diets will advise that you take time each day to perform a complete body cleansing. There are several ways to aid your detox diet plan, whether it's with herbs, baths or saunas. Some diets even suggest laxatives or enemas to help the process along. Now that you know what a basic detox diet plan involves, you might be curious to find out exactly what kinds of foods are permitted. Anyone looking to follow a detox diet plan must consult a nutritionist before getting started on it. The following plan is an example of what can be followed on the first day of a 3-day diet plan.There are lots of different definitions of what defines the best detox diet or the best cleanse for weight loss. However, a good detox diet should supply all of the important nutrients that your body needs while also cutting out the chemicals, junk and added ingredients that it doesn't. Following a few easy guidelines and incorporating some detox foods into your diet is the best way to optimize your built-in detox system and supply your liver with the tools it needs to clear out toxins efficiently. Wondering how to detox your body without spending a fortune on expensive programs and products? Luckily, following a detox diet for weight loss and better health can be as simple as making a few simple swaps in your diet. Here are some of the basic rules to follow on a healthy detox diet:

Switch out sugar-sweetened beverages like sodas and sports drinks for water, unsweetened tea or detox drinks, and be sure to stay well-hydrated.

Nix added sugars from your diet from foods like candies, cakes, cookies and sweets, and aim for a sugar-free diet instead.

Cut out all heavily processed and refined foods, such as convenience meals, pre-packaged snacks, and store-bought cakes and cookies.

Up your intake of whole ingredients and raw foods, including fruits, veggies, healthy protein foods and whole grains.

Swap processed meats like bacon, hot dogs and sausages for better options, such as grass-fed beef, wild-caught salmon and organic chicken. If you're following a vegetarian or vegan diet, there are also plenty of plant-based protein foods available, including nuts, seeds and legumes.

Include more natural detox foods in your diet, such as grapefruit, bone broth, Brussels sprouts, berries, beets, chia seeds and nuts.

Trade in your salt shaker for some healing herbs and spices instead. Seasonings like cumin, basil, parsley and paprika can bump up the flavor of your foods while also providing a host of powerful health benefits.

Adjust your sleep schedule to ensure you're squeezing in at least eight hours per night, which allows your body to heal and restore.

 Get in some daily exercise, and stay active with your favorite workouts, such as walking, jogging or biking.

Minimize your stress levels and incorporate some natural stress relievers into your routine, such as yoga, meditation, journaling and essential oils.

Whether you decide to do a three-day detox diet, a five-day detox diet plan or a full seven-day cleanse diet, you have plenty of options for delicious and healthy foods to enjoy. Use the meal pattern below to get some ideas, and feel free to follow the plan as long as you'd like to jump-start your detox.

Day One

Breakfast: Egg white omelette with tomatoes, garlic, onions and peppers + 1 banana

Snack: Omega blueberry smoothie

Lunch: Baked chicken with broccoli and brown rice

Snack: Walnuts and dried fruit

Dinner: Chickpea and veggie stew + roasted Brussels sprouts

Day Two

Breakfast: Raw yogurt with chia seeds and fresh fruit + grainless granola

Snack: Carrots with hummus

Lunch: Roasted salmon with zucchini and baked sweet potato

Snack: Cottage cheese with celery and tomatoes

Dinner: Portobello mushroom pizza with arugula salad

Day Three

Breakfast: 2 hard-boiled eggs + whole wheat toast with avocado

Snack: Apple slices topped with cinnamon and raw honey

Lunch: Quinoa and veggie stuffed bell peppers

Snack: Almond butter banana protein bar

Dinner: Grilled chicken, avocado and grapefruit salad

Day Four

Breakfast: Paleo protein pancakes + fresh fruit

Snack: Dark chocolate with sliced strawberries

Lunch: Turkey burger in lettuce wrap with sautéed veggies

Snack: Chia seed pudding with strawberries and rhubarb

Dinner: Sweet potato hash with black beans and spinach

Day Five

Breakfast: Overnight oatmeal with berries, nuts and cinnamon

Snack: Baked apple chips

Lunch: Steak and Brussels sprouts stir-fry

Snack: Energy balls

Dinner: Marinated tempeh with herbed garlic lentils

Day Six

Breakfast: Broiled grapefruit with raw honey and bananas + kale and feta egg bake

Snack: Gut-healing smoothie

Lunch: Greek meatballs with orzo pilaf

Snack: Garlic roasted chickpeas

Dinner: Pulled beef sliders with carrot chips

Day Seven

Breakfast: Sweet potato toast topped with avocado and fried egg

Snack: Air-popped popcorn

Lunch: Mediterranean grilled lamb chops with cauliflower tabbouleh

Snack: Almonds with blueberries

Dinner: Lemon chicken with roasted Brussels sprouts

Since the whole point of a detox diet is to eliminate all of your body's harmful toxins, there are certain foods that are either allowed or shunned. Many foods that we consume on a regular basis can be clouded with toxins such as pesticides, mercury and food additives. Other things you would want to stay away from are alcohol, caffeine, tobacco, drugs, refined or overly processed food and supplements that have too many additives. Detox Diet Foods Since the whole point of a detox diet is to eliminate all of your body's harmful toxins, there are certain foods that are either allowed or shunned. Many foods that we consume on a regular basis can be clouded with toxins such as pesticides, mercury and food additives. Other things you would want to stay away from are alcohol, caffeine, tobacco, drugs, refined or overly processed food and supplements that have too many additives.

Best Detox Foods

Grapefruit

Brussels Sprouts

Berries

Beets

Chia Seeds

Nuts

Bone Broth

Grapefruit

This tasty citrus fruit is well-known for its multitude of health-promoting properties, especially when it comes to detoxification. According to a 2005 animal model out of Israel, grapefruit juice was found to be incredibly effective in bumping up the levels of liver enzymes involved in detoxification. (1) Including a serving or two of grapefruit or grapefruit juice in your diet each day can be a simple way to keep your liver healthy and support its natural detox abilities.

Brussels Sprouts

Hearty, flavorful and full of fiber, Brussels sprouts make an awesome addition to a healthy detox diet. Not only can they promote regularity to get things moving, but Brussels sprouts have also been shown to boost liver health and enhance detoxification. In fact, one study published in Carcinogenesis showed that eating just 300 grams of Brussels sprouts daily was able to amp up the levels of detox enzymes by a whopping 30 percent.

Berries

Besides being delicious and incredibly versatile, berries are a great source of both fiber and antioxidants, two important components of a well-balanced detox diet. Fiber moves slowly through the gastrointestinal tract and helps bulk up the stool to support regularity and excrete waste more efficiently. Antioxidants, on the other hand, have been shown in animal models to protect the liver against oxidative stress while simultaneously preserving immune cell function. Berries like blueberries and strawberries also have a high water content and can promote hydration as well as proper elimination.

Beets

There are plenty of reasons to consider adding beets to your diet. Not only are they vibrant and full of color, but they're also high in an array of vitamins, minerals and micronutrients that can boost detoxification. One animal study found that drinking beetroot juice regularly helped increase the levels of several key enzymes involved in detoxification. Similarly, another animal study published in the Journal of Agricultural and Food Chemistry showed that beetroot juice decreased lipid peroxidation, a marker used to measure cell damage, in the liver by 38 percent.

Chia Seeds

Frequently touted as a superfood, chia seed benefits range from enhanced digestion to better blood sugar control. Not surprisingly, chia seeds may also aid in detoxification as well. They pack in tons of fiber, which can help keep things moving through the digestive system, allowing waste products to be excreted efficiently. Plus, they're high in antioxidants to fight off free radicals and protect your liver against damage and disease.

Nuts

It's no secret that nuts are great for your health. They're high in fiber, antioxidants, protein, heart-healthy fats as well as an assortment of the key vitamins and minerals that your body needs to stay healthy. In addition to keeping you regular due to their high fiber content, including healthy nuts in your diet can also help optimize liver function as well. Studies show that eating more nuts is linked to a lower risk of non-alcoholic fatty liver disease as well as enhanced liver enzyme levels to maximize your body's detoxifying potential.

Bone Broth

Bone broth, a liquid made from the water left over after simmering bones for up to a day at a time, has been associated with a number of incredible benefits. Perhaps most impressive, however, is its potent effects on detoxification. Studies suggest that bone broth may help improve immune health by reducing inflammation, allowing your body to work more effectively at removing harmful toxins, bacteria and pathogens from the body. Because it's rich in collagen and an assortment of amino acids, it's also believed to help seal the gut and protect against leaky gut syndrome, a condition that allows toxins and particles to seep from the gut into the bloodstream.

In order to remove the toxins from the body, detox diet is used. In order to use the methods there are some points that have to be kept in mind. First and foremost, detox diet does not help in shedding of weight. It only helps in the flushing out of toxins from the system and cleaning the system. While following the detox diet, one has to pertain from consuming some types of food, and have laxatives in order to clean the liver and intestine. During the detox diet program, one needs to eat an extra amount of vegetables and fruits, preferably raw, because processed and cooked food have lesser amount of minerals and vitamins. People who took this diet claim to feel better and much healthier and energetic. People suffering from eating disorders, diabetes, heart diseases or any other problems should not even consider taking this diet. Also pregnant or nursing women should refrain from this diet. It?s anytime better to take the doctor's advice before starting the diet regime. This diet should be avoided by teenagers as it may refrain them from certain vital minerals and vitamins which are necessary during the growth phase.

How frequent?

One should go for a detox diet once or may be twice in a year only. It should not become a frequent habit as it then may become as an addiction, people tend to get addicted to it as they get addicted to drugs and smoking.

People getting addicted, find it very hard to come out of it and eventually develop heart diseases or eating disorders or sometimes may even die. Even though detox diet is healthy, it also comes with its share of side effects such as headache, hunger, acne, petulance and hunger. These conditions are also experienced when you have detox supplements because they also are laxatives. Visits to the bathroom may become very often and that sometimes becomes a messy and embarrassing affair. Other effects are deficiency of water that leads to dehydration, loss of minerals and many more digestive disorders. In order to prevent these conditions it is necessary to drink lots of water while dieting.

The point to remember here is that loss of muscles and water during detox diet does not mean weight loss. Once the program ends and the normal diet are restarted, everything lost is regained.

So just like everything, detox diet also has its share of plus points and negative points. Now that you have the knowledge, you can decide accordingly whether to take the diet or leave it. It is still advisable to take your doctor's advice before starting the diet.

Other than detox diets, there is other programs too for cleaning the system. One program that works for a person may not for another. So it is better to do under the doctor's supervision.

How to begin a detox diet?

We've worked across why one should take on such a diet. The

following steps might help in beginning your detox diet:

The first thing to do before starting is to consult a nutritionist or a doctor. Ensure that following this diet will not cause any detrimental effects on your health.

Prepare to give up stimulants such as caffeine, alcohol, or tobacco. Replace them with lemon water, infused or herbal tea, or simply water.

Choose a type of detox diet that suits you the best. The diet varies from person to person based on their physique and general calorie intake.

Removal of toxins can cause symptoms like nausea, headaches, and vomiting, which are temporary and occur in the initial stages. Prepare yourself for such situations.

Plan your detox such that you don't completely stop eating solid food. This is because; a pure detox

diet does not contain
carbohydrates or proteins which
your body needs. So, make sure
that you are getting enough
nutrition but in a healthier way.

Prepare for headaches, tiredness,
and nausea, which usually occur in
the initial stages.

Avoid exercise during a detox. Your
body has a decreased calorie
intake, so, exercising is not
beneficial during the course of this
diet. It can cause tiredness and
fatigue.

It is possible that during this diet, your tongue may get coated. Use a tongue scraper to remove this layer of bacteria.

You can definitely consume fruit and vegetables if you are looking to improve gut health as such foods contain fiber.

After the detox is over, and if you have not consumed solid foods during the course, ensure that you re-introduce it slowly but surely. If you suddenly begin eating solid food, your system will be disturbed.

For a juice diet:

Try to use organic fruits and vegetables.

Try to make your juices at home rather than buying packaged ones as they may contain preservatives and excess sugar, which goes against the purpose of your diet.

Try to use the whole fruit, including the peel while juicing. This is because; the peel also contains a lot of nutrients and minerals which are beneficial for the body.

Try to consume all your juice immediately after you have made them. Storing juices is not recommended.

Furthermore, consume fruits that are low on the glycemic index, i.e., use low sugar fruits. Although you may not like the taste of some green vegetables, those contain the most nutrients.

You can certainly try to improve the taste of your juices by adding flavorsome herbs or other spices.

Moreover, try your best to use locally grown produce to enjoy good taste and even better nutrition.

Ensure that you are hydrated throughout your diet. It is absolutely necessary to drink lots of water as it flushes out toxins.

How to Successfully Undergo a Detox Diet

You may have been enticed to attempt the detox diet after a few actresses highlighted over the TV how it has helped them to lose weight. Yes, it is possible to lose weight utilizing the detox program and you too can do it successfully as long as you keep in mind some basic things. Before starting on the diet, counsel your specialist on whether it is safe for you. Pregnant and nursing ladies must not undertake this eating regimen, nor should individuals with diabetes, heart sicknesses or other chronic conditions. Before you really start counting calories, you need to prepare your body for it. Stop taking nicotine, caffeine, alcohol, sugar and certain food at least a week prior to going on the diet. Drink lots of water and have enough rest. Exercise for at least 20 to 30 minutes every day before undertaking the diet. This prepares your body physically for what is to come. Exercise even during and after the diet is over, to boost your energy level. Buy plenty of organic products before embarking on the diet. Ideally organic ones. Be that as it may in the event that you can't get them, even normal ones will do, provided you peel off the skin and wash the natural products well before consuming. All detox diets do not require you to have raw food. There are certain consumes less calories in which you need to eat cooked vegetables partially-say 15% cooked and 85% raw. So that you are not bored of eating the equivalent food again and again, you may introduce variations by mixing a couple of couple of them together. However, for that, you need to know which ones of them go together. Try mixing tomatoes or carrots with celery, spinach or cucumber, or if it is organic products you are experimenting with, use apple, cranberry or pineapple together, yet don't use oranges as they are very acidic. Juices are supportive as well, however on the off chance that you can't get them, a regular mixed is fine. Have at least 64 ounces of fruits and vegetables, and 6-8 glasses of water everyday for the term of the diet. On the off chance that you couldnt finish the beverage the day you made it, don't fret. Fruit juices stay well for

3 days, while vegetable ones will last for 5 days. On the off chance that the detox program endures longer, say for 3 days or more, eat some solid food in the succeeding days. In the event that you feel nauseous, or lightheaded, or have the tendency to throw up anytime during the program, it's best to stop the diet, consult the specialist, and continue the program just if the specialist approves of it. When you are over with the diet, switch back to strong food. Detox diets are good only for short term, and prolonging them may result in terrible health. In the event that

you are happy with the results of the eating regimen, you can take up the diet again, however don?t do it more frequently, than once or twice a year.Apart from cleaning up your system, detox diet has the added effect of helping you lose weight. But don?t be fooled, as what you have lost is only water, which you'll regain very soon when you take up the normal diet. There are plenty of detox diets you can choose from. Read about each one to know about them. If you don't like to drink it, you also have the choice to eat it.

How Effective Are These Diets?

Some people report feeling more focused and energetic during and after detox diets. However, this improved well-being may simply be due to eliminating processed foods, alcohol, and other unhealthy substances from your diet. You may also be getting vitamins and minerals that were lacking before. That said, many people also report feeling very unwell during the detox period.

Effects on Weight Loss

Very few scientific studies have investigated how detox diets impact weight loss. While some people may lose a lot of weight quickly, this effect seems to be due to loss of fluid and carb stores rather than fat. This weight is usually regained quickly once you go off the cleanse. One study in overweight Korean women examined the lemon detox diet, which limits you to a mixture of organic maple or palm syrups and lemon juice for seven days. This diet significantly reduced body weight, BMI, body fat percentage, waist-to-hip ratio, waist circumference, markers of inflammation, insulin resistance, and circulating leptin levels. If a detox diet involves severe calorie restriction, it will most certainly cause weight loss and improvements in metabolic health — but it's unlikely to help you keep weight off in the long term.

Detox Diets, Short-Term Fasting, and Stress

Several varieties of detox diets may have effects similar to those of short-term or intermittent fasting. Short-term fasting may improve various disease markers in some people, including improved leptin and insulin sensitivity. However, these effects do not apply to everyone. Studies in women show that both a 48-hour fast and a 3-week period of reduced calorie intake may increase your stress hormone levels. On top of that, crash diets can be a stressful experience, as they involve resisting temptations and feeling extreme hunger.

A few aspects of detox diets may have health benefits, such as:

Avoiding dietary sources of heavy metals and POPs

Losing excessive fat

Exercising and sweating regularly

Eating whole, nutritious, healthy foods

Avoiding processed foods

Drinking water and green tea

Limiting stress, relaxing, and getting good sleep

Safety and Side Effects

Before doing any sort of detox, it is important to consider possible side effects.

Severe Calorie Restriction

Several detox diets recommend fasting or severe calorie restriction. Short-term fasting and limited calorie intake can result in fatigue, irritability, and bad breath.

Long-term fasting can result in energy, vitamin, and mineral deficiencies, as well as electrolyte imbalance and even death.

Furthermore, colon cleansing methods, which are sometimes recommended during detoxes, can cause dehydration, cramping, bloating, nausea, and vomiting.

Overdosing

Some detox diets may pose the risk of overdosing on supplements, laxatives, diuretics, and even water.

There is a lack of regulation and monitoring in the detox industry, and many detox foods and supplements may not have any scientific basis.

In the worst cases, the ingredient labels of detox products may be inaccurate. This can increase your risk of overdosing, potentially resulting in serious — and even fatal — effects.

At-Risk Populations

Certain people should not start any detox or calorie-restricting regimens without consulting a doctor first. At-risk populations include children, adolescents, older adults, those who are malnourished, pregnant or lactating women, and people who have blood sugar issues, such as diabetes or an eating disorder.

Natural detox mechanisms

The body itself has numerous ways of removing toxins on its own. The body eliminates its toxins through urine, through sweat, through the kidneys, the liver, the immune system, and the respiratory system. Therefore, these mechanisms of the body render the idea of detoxification to be completely redundant. The body does not allow toxins to get accumulated, so there is nothing to "de-toxify," which the diet claims to do.

Should You Be On The Detox Diet If You Are On Medication?

A detox diet is all about eating clean and incorporating healthy habits to promote better health. Hence, you can be on a detox diet while you are on medication. But always check with your doctor before starting the diet plan.

Cucumber and Ginger Detox Smoothie

This smoothie with ginger and cucumber is great for your digestive system! It also contains oranges which is a great source of vitamin C.

Ingredients

30g spinach

1 cucumber

1 orange

1/2 avocado

1/2 inch ginger

1 cup of water

1 cup ice

Direction

Chop the cucumbers and the
ginger.

Peel the oranges

Cut the avocado in half and scoop
it out.

Wash the spinach leaves
thoroughly and roughly chop them

Add all the ingredients into a blender along with water

Blend the ingredients together until there are no lumps. Serve

Yellow Turmeric Ginger Smoothie

This smoothie has the detoxifying properties of both turmeric and ginger! This also contains squash which is a great source of iron, magnesium, and folate!

Ingredients

1 yellow squash

1 orange

1/2 tsp turmeric

1/2 inch ginger

1 tbsp hemp seed

1 cup of water

1 cup ice

Direction

Chop the squash into small pieces.

Peel the orange and chop the ginger

Add all the ingredients into a blender

Add water and blend until smooth. Serve

Lemon Cucumber Mint Detox Water

Ingredients

6 cups water

3 large lemons

1 1 large English cucumber, sliced
or 4 small Persian cucumbers,
sliced

8 sprigs mint

ice

Direction

Fill up a pitcher with water (about
6 cups). Squeeze the juice from 2

lemons into the pitcher. Cut the third lemon into slices and it to the pitcher along with cucumber slices and mint and let all ingredients set for 1-3 hours before drinking. The longer it sets the more flavorful the water. Fill the remaining pitcher with ice. Enjoy chilled in a glass.

Apple Cider Vinegar Weight Loss Drink

Ingredients

1 cup water

1 tablespoon apple cider vinegar

3 tablespoons lemon juice
(optional to reserve slices to add to
the water)

liquid Stevia few drops to sweeten
to desired taste, or 1 tablespoon
maple syrup or honey

Direction

In a glass add ice, water, apple
cider vinegar, lemon juice and a
few drops of liquid Stevia (or 1
tablespoon of maple syrup or
honey) to sweeten to desired
taste. Mix well and enjoy! Or skip
the ice and drink warm for best
absorption.

Orange And Ginger Detox Drink

Ingredients

1 Large carrot

2 Oranges

1/2 inch raw turmeric (crushed)

1/2 inch ginger (crushed)

1/2 Lemon (juiced)

Direction

Juice the orange and carrot
separately.

Pour the juice in a blender add
turmeric and ginger.

Blend for 30 seconds and then
squeeze half lemon.

Strain and serve.

Ingredients

5 Lemons whole

3 Bunch Mint

1/2 Cup Honey

Crushed ice

Direction

Blitz all the ingredients along with lots of crushed ice in a blender and serve chilled.

Cucumber Mint Detox Drink

Another summery delight, another reason to rejoice! Mint is traditionally regarded as the best ingredients for soothing an upset stomach. Mint also improves the flow of bile through the stomach speeding the digestion process.

Coupled with antioxidant rich cucumber and lemon, this cooler is as much a respite from the bustling heat as from the toxic overload. cucumber mint cooler

Ingredients:

1 Cucumber

8-10 Mint leaves

2 Tbsp Lemon juice

Ice cubes

Iced Water

Lemon rings and mint leaves

Instructions:

Peel, chop and blend cucumber, mint leaves and 1 cup of water.

Strain and discard pulp.

Add lemon juice, black salt and
dilute with water if needed.

Pour the beverages in glasses, put
some ice cubes and garnish with
lemon rings and mint leaves

Pomegranate Juice

Detox with the goodness of
pomegranate and beetroot that
are also given immense
importance in Ayurveda for its
umpteen cleansing and detox

benefits. The fresh aloe vera gel used in the juice gives further boost to your immunity system.

Ingredients

1 Fresh leaf aloe vera

1/2 cup Beetroot, chopped

2 cups Pomegranate juice or amla juice (Indian gooseberry)

1/4 tsp Black pepper powder

Direction

Take a sharp knife and carefully peel the rind from the aloe vera plant leaves and discard the rind.2.Peel the yellow layer

just beneath the rind with a sharp knife and you should be left with approximately 2 Tbsp (30 ml) of clear aloe vera gel. (Clean the gel before adding to the juice.)

In a blender add pomegranate
juice, chopped beetroot and blend.

Now add aloe vera gel. Give it a
whiz.

Lastly add some black pepper and
serve.

A lemon water detox is one of the best detox drinks recommended by fitness enthusiasts to shed those extra kilos being rich in pectin fibre. This fibre gives you the feeling of fullness for a long period of time and thus delays hunger. This recipe is also infused with the goodness of carrots, apples, beetroot and radish.

Ingredients

1 apple, chopped

1 carrot, chopped

1/2 beetroot, sliced

2-3 slices white radish

1/2 tsp lemon zest

2 lemons (juiced)

Direction

Mix all the ingredients in a blender.

Add little bit of water to adjust the consistency.

Sieve and serve.

India and its love for tea requires no introduction. Spiced with a hint of ginger, honey and lemon, this drink has long been used to treat sore throats and cold. But the concoction packs more benefits than you thought.

Ingredients

3 Cups Water

1 tsp Ginger, finely chopped

1 tsp Tea leaves, for every cup

1 tsp Lemon juice

1 tsp Honey

Direction

In a pan heat 3 cups of water.

Before it begins to boil add ginger.

Just as it starts to boil add the tea leaves, lemon juice and honey.

Strain it into a cup and enjoy!

Healthy Detox Smoothie

The detox smoothie is refreshing and nutrient dense. Detox smoothie flushes out the harmful toxins and makes the skin glow. It is rich in fiber, vitamin A, K and potassium. This smoothie helps prevent cravings for junk foods and keeps hunger at bay.

Ingredients:

1/2 Green apple Spinach leaves 1/2 cup

Pineapple juice 150 ml

Avocado 1/4 cup

Broccoli florets 4 to 5

Direction:

Blend all the ingredients in a blender until smooth.

Refrigerate if required and serve.

Conclusion

Your body is often exposed to toxic substances. However, most of the time, it can remove them without additional help. While detox eats less may seem enticing, their advantages probably have nothing to do with vanquishing toxins, yet rather with eliminating various unhealthy foods. A much smarter approach is to eat healthier and improve your lifestyle rather than go on a possibly perilous purify. Following a detox diet can help give your body with the nutrients that it needs to be ready to clear out toxins effectively. Although there are plenty of regimens and detox programs out there, the best detox scrub is one that gives your body what it needs instead of denying it of important vitamins and minerals. Several foods have additionally been shown to help detox your body and enhance the work of your built-in detox system to keep you sound. Cutting out garbage, increasing your intake of whole foods and following a healthy lifestyle can help your body detoxify more efficiently.